The Ultimate Cancer Diet

Cookbook For Newly Diagnosed Individuals

25 Healing Recipes to Empower, Nourish, and Support Those Newly Diagnosed with Cancer on Their Journey to a Long and Healthy Life

Rose V Allen

About the Author

Meet the passionate author behind the "The Ultimate Cancer Diet Cookbook for Newly Diagnosed Individuals ," Rose V Allen. A proud U.S. native, Rose is a dedicated advocate for health and nutrition. Armed with a second-class upper degree in nutritional Biochemistry from Harvard State University, her educational journey laid the foundation for a career driven by a commitment to wellness.

With extensive experience in the field of nutrition and health, Rose brings a unique blend of expertise and a deep understanding of the challenges faced by those managing cancer. Fueled by a passion for empowering individuals to take control of their health, she crafted this cookbook as a comprehensive guide to restoring, nourishing, and protecting cancer from peoples.

Rose combines her academic knowledge with practical insights gained from years of working in a clinic as a nutritionist. Her mission is to make a positive impact on the lives of individuals managing cancer by providing not just recipes, but a holistic approach to health and well-being. The "The Ultimate Cancer Diet Cookbook for Newly Diagnosed Individuals" reflects her dedication to merging culinary delights with science-backed strategies for cancer control and health preservation.

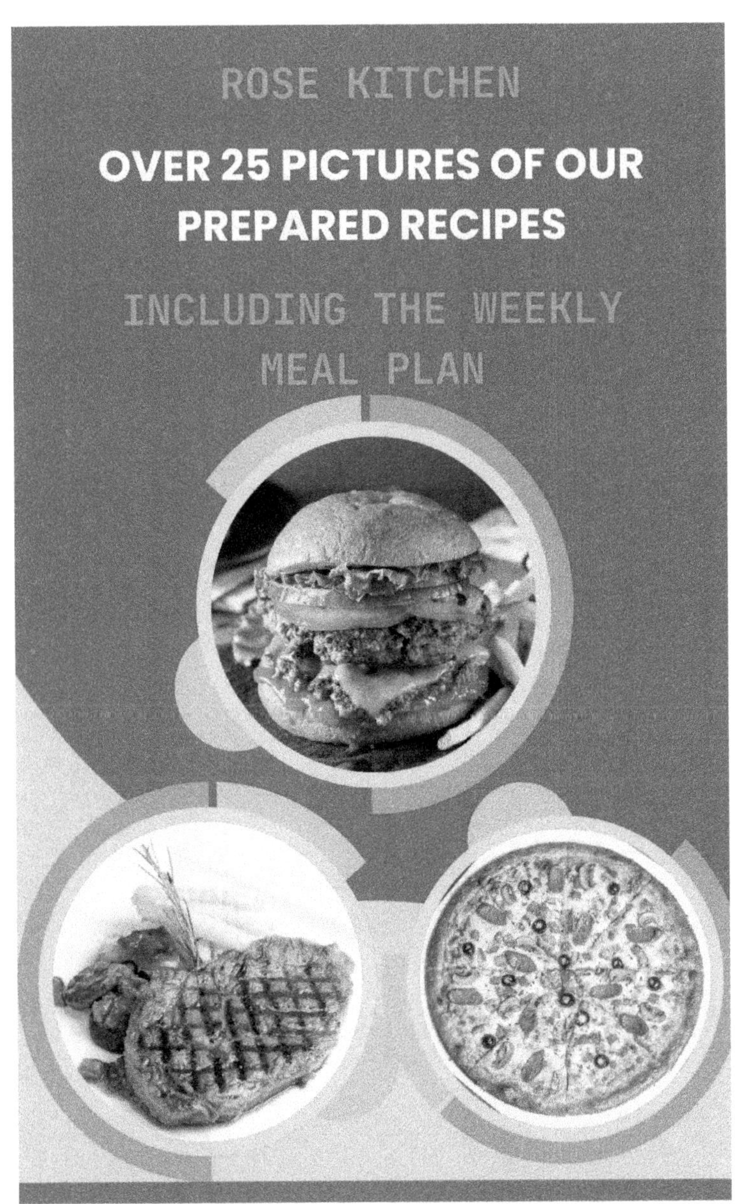

ROSE KITCHEN
OVER 25 PICTURES OF OUR
PREPARED RECIPES
INCLUDING THE WEEKLY
MEAL PLAN

INTRODUCTION

Here you will find "The Ultimate Cancer Diet Cookbook for Newly Diagnosed Individuals"—a path to recovery, strength, and delicious new recipes. To those who are dealing with the complicated range of feelings brought on by a cancer diagnosis, our deepest sympathies are with you in this moving introduction.

We hope that you will find this cookbook to be more than just a resource; rather, it will be a reassuring friend as you work towards healing. It is with deepest sympathy that we offer our assistance as you face the mental and physical obstacles brought on by a cancer diagnosis.

We take a moment to recognize the critical role that nutrition plays in your recovery journey in the flurry of medical therapies.

Even outside of the confines of the hospital, at the very core of your house, you have an ally—your kitchen.

We believe in building your physical and mental resilience via purposeful, wholesome meals, which feed your body and spirit.

The inspiration for this cookbook comes from my battle with cancer, so please allow me to share a little bit of my story. During my journey through treatment and recovery, I came to realise the immense impact that healing meals can have on one's life. Not only is it a collection of recipes, but it is also a representation of the lessons and optimism that I have learned from my own experience with cancer.

The motive for developing this cookbook is profoundly personal. It arises from a desire to transmit not only recipes but a feeling of empowerment, a culinary toolset that nurtures strength, and a testimony to the conviction that what we place on our plates can be a source of healing and rejuvenation.

Mission and Approach

Our aim is clear—to inspire, nurture, and encourage those who find themselves at the crossroads of a cancer diagnosis. Through these pages, we welcome you to embark on a holistic path toward healing, embracing the connection of mind, body, and spirit.

Beyond the traditional knowledge of nutrition, our approach is comprehensive. It's about knowing that healing is not restricted to one part of life but embraces every dimension of your existence. The dishes offered in this cookbook are not only about food; they are about generating moments of nourishment and pleasure amid tough situations.

In "The Ultimate Cancer Diet Cookbook," we don't simply supply recipes; we provide a hand to grasp, a source of strength, and a light of hope. This is more than a cookbook; it's a monument to the transformational power of food, community, and perseverance. Welcome to a journey where each page is a step towards a long and healthy life, filled with hope, healing, and great food.

CHAPTER ONE

Nourishing Resilience - Unlocking the Healing Power of Nutrition

Overview of Nutrition and Cancer:

In this revolutionary chapter, we dig into the fundamental relationship between nutrition and the body's incredible capacity to battle and conquer the obstacles offered by cancer. Picture your body as a robust castle, strengthened by the decisions you make in the kitchen. We uncover the complicated dance between nutrition and healing, exposing how a well-crafted diet may stand as a steadfast friend in your battle against cancer.

The Impact of Nutrition:

Embark on a voyage of discovery as we shed light on the crucial role nutrition plays in not only strengthening your body but also boosting your intellect. The nutrients you pick become more than simply nutrition; they become agents of strength, boosting your body's inherent defenses. Together, we study the interesting science underlying how appropriate nutrition may boost the efficacy of medical therapies, paving the road for a more robust recovery.

Complementing Medical Treatments:

Imagine your body as a symphony, with medical therapies as the conductor directing the struggle against cancer. Here, we illustrate how a well-balanced diet takes on the role of the supporting ensemble, harmonizing with medical procedures to produce a thorough and powerful healing song.

This is not only about what you eat; it's about coordinating a holistic strategy that addresses every area of your well-being.

Nutritional Needs for Newly Diagnosed Individuals:

As we explore further into the chapter, we uncover the subtleties of dietary needs designed particularly for patients navigating the early phases of cancer therapy. We give a roadmap, a nutritional compass to lead you through the maze of food choices, ensuring that every mouthful adds to your vitality.

Specific Nutritional Requirements:

With an emphasis on accuracy, we detail the particular nutrients your body demands during this important moment. From immune-boosting antioxidants to energy-packed staples, each suggestion is a carefully picked building stone based on your recovery. This area is a treasure mine of knowledge, helping you to make educated decisions that connect with your body's specific requirements.

Addressing Concerns and Misconceptions:

In this instructive section, we face prevalent fears and misunderstandings regarding the link between nutrition and cancer. We clarify misconceptions, alleviate worries, and give clarity on the nutritional choices that may be a source of strength. Your trip is a customized tale, and we guarantee that your queries find solutions inside these pages.

In "Nourishing Resilience," Chapter 1 is not simply an introduction; it's a doorway to a comprehensive knowledge of the synergistic link between nutrition and cancer recovery. As you browse these pages, imagine each piece of advice as a stepping stone towards a fortified and empowered you - a witness to the transforming potential of mindful eating in your recovery path.

Cancer is a disorder in which some of the body's cells grow uncontrolled and spread to other parts of the body.

Cancer may begin nearly anywhere in the body of a person, which is comprised of billions of cells. Normally, human cells grow and proliferate (by a process called cell division) to make new cells whenever the body demands them. When cells get old or become harmed they die, and fresh cells take their place.

Sometimes this controlled process goes down, and abnormal or damaged cells grow and multiply when they should not. These cells may become tumors, which are lumps of tissue. Carcinoma may be cancerous or noncancerous (benign).

Cancerous tumours spread into, or invade, surrounding tissues and may travel to distant locations in the body to generate new tumours (a process called metastasis).

Cancerous tumors might also be termed carcinogenic tumors.

Many cancers produce solid tumors, but malignancies of the blood, such as leukemias, generally do not.

Benign tumors do not expand into, or invade, adjacent tissues. When removed, benign tumors typically don't come back, while malignant ones rarely do. Benign tumors may sometimes be exceedingly huge, however. Some may generate serious symptoms or be life-threatening, such as benign tumours in the brain.

How Cancer develops

Cancer is a genetic disease—that is, it is caused by mutations to genes that govern the way our cells behave, especially how they grow and divide.

Genetic changes that cause cancer may originate because of errors that occur when cells multiply.

of DNA damage caused by hazardous substances in the environment, such as the poisons in tobacco smoke and UV rays from the sun. (Our Cancer Causes and Prevention section includes extra information.)

they were inherited from our parents.

The body normally eliminates cells with damaged DNA before they grow cancerous. But the body's power to do so becomes lessened as we age. This is part of the reason why there is an increased risk of cancer later in life.

Each person's cancer has a unique combination of genetic changes. As the cancer continues to progress, more abnormalities will occur. Even within the same tumour, individual cells may have diverse genetic changes.

How it spread

A cancer that has migrated from the spot where it first formed to another region in the body is called metastatic cancer. The process by which cancer cells travel to different parts of the body is called metastasis.

Metastatic cancer has the same name and the same kind of cancer cells as the first, or primary, cancer.

For example, breast cancer that develops an aggressive tumor in the lung is spreading breast cancer, not lung cancer.

Under a microscope, metastatic cancer cells typically resemble the same cells of the underlying tumour. Moreover, metastatic cancer cells and cells of the primary malignancy typically have specific genetic properties in common, such as the presence of certain chromosomal abnormalities.

In some instances, treatment may help prolong the lives of patients with metastatic cancer. In other instances, the major purpose of treatment for metastatic cancer is to control the course of the illness or to relieve symptoms it is causing. Metastatic tumors may cause severe damage to how the body operates, and most individuals who die of cancer die of metastatic sickness.

Types of Cancer

Breast Cancer:

Breast cancer occurs in the cells of the breast, often in the ducts or lobules. It may occur in both males and women, yet it is more frequent in women. Breast cancer is often characterized by the presence of a lump or abnormalities in the breast tissue.

Lung Cancer:

Lung cancer develops in the lungs and may occur in both the small cells and the non-small cells of the lung tissue. Smoking is a considerable risk factor for lung cancer, however, non-smokers may also acquire the condition.

Colorectal Cancer:

Colorectal cancer encompasses malignancies of the gut and rectum.It frequently begins as polyps, abnormal growths in the lining of the colon or rectum, which may become malignant over time. Early diagnosis via screenings is crucial for effective treatment.

Prostate Cancer:

Prostate cancer arises in the prostate, a small organ that produces seminal fluid in men. It is one of the most prevalent cancers among guys. Prostate cancer may progress slowly, and certain occurrences may not require quick treatment.

Ovarian Cancer:

Ovarian cancer arises in the ovaries, the female reproductive organs responsible for generating eggs and hormones. It is frequently harder to recognize in the early stages, leading to a larger probability of advanced disease upon diagnosis.

Pancreatic Cancer:

Pancreatic cancer occurs in the pancreas, an organ that aids in digesting and managing blood sugar. It is often identified at an advanced stage, making it harder to treat. Smoking, genetics, and permanent pancreatitis are risk factors.

Leukaemia:

Leukaemia is a kind of cancer affecting the blood cells and bone marrow. It involves the overproduction of aberrant white blood cells, inhibiting the production of healthy ones. Leukemia may be acute or chronic and is graded based on the sort of blood cell involved.

Lymphoma:

Lymphoma is a tumour of the lymphatic system, which includes lymph nodes, spleen, thymus, and bone marrow.

hodgkin's lymphoma, which is and other types of lymphoma are the two basic forms.

it commonly presents as enlarged lymph nodes and might weaken the body's defenses

melanoma:

Melanoma is a sort of skin cancer that develops in the pigment-producing cells (melanocytes). It is renowned for its potential to spread fast to other regions of the body. Early detection and protection against UV radiation are crucial for prevention.

Cervical Cancer:

Cervical cancer occurs in the cervix, the lower portion of the uterus. Persistent infection with some strains of human papillomavirus (HPV) is a substantial risk factor for cervical cancer. Regular testing, such as Pap smears, may help spot precancerous abnormalities.

Main causes of cancer

Cancer is a wide group of disorders, and its causes are different. While the precise causes could differ depending on the sort of cancer, there are common elements related to the development of cancer. Here is a summary of some of the important causes:

Genetic Factors:

Inherited genetic changes may predispose individuals to certain kinds of cancer. These mutations may be carried on from parents to their offspring and may boost the risk of cancer development.

Environmental Factors:

Exposure to certain environmental components, such as carcinogens (cancer-causing substances), may contribute to the development of cancer.

Examples include tobacco smoke, asbestos, pollution, and certain chemicals.

Lifestyle Choices:

Unhealthy lifestyle choices are associated with an increased risk of cancer. Factors such as smoking, excessive alcohol use, a poor diet rich in processed foods, lack of physical activity, and obesity have been connected with higher cancer risks.

Age:

The risk of cancer typically grows with age. As cells divide over time, errors in the replication process may accumulate, potentially leading to malignant cell growth.

Immunosuppression:

A weakened immune system may fail to detect and eliminate abnormal cells, causing them to develop and form tumours.

Conditions such as HIV/AIDS and several medicines that affect the immune system could boost cancer risk.

Chronic Inflammation:

Persistent inflammation, typically occurring from persistent infections or disorders such as inflammatory bowel disease, may contribute to the development of cancer. Inflammatory activity may damage DNA and promote the formation of cancer cells.

Hormonal Factors:

Hormonal imbalances or chronic exposure to certain hormones may affect the probability of contracting different cancers. For example, hormonal changes during menstruation, pregnancy, or hormone replacement medication may raise breast and ovarian cancer risks.

Radiation Exposure:

Exposure to ionising radiation, which is whether from therapeutic techniques (such as radiation therapy) or the environment (such as UV rays from the sun), may damage DNA and elevate the risk of cancer.

Infections:

Some infections caused by viruses, bacteria, or protozoa have been connected to an increased risk of cancer. Examples include human papillomavirus (HPV) and cancer of the cervical region, Helicobacter pylori and stomach cancer, and hepatitis B or C viruses and liver cancer.

Occupational Hazards:

Some jobs require exposure to harmful substances, such as asbestos, benzene, or certain chemicals, which may lead to a higher risk of contracting cancer.

It's vital to highlight that while these factors could boost the risk of cancer, they do not assure its development. Many cancers emerge from a combination of genetic predisposition and environmental influences. Adopting a healthy lifestyle, regular checkups, and avoiding identified risk factors may drastically lessen the probability of cancer.

Symptoms of cancer

The symptoms of cancer may vary widely depending on the sort of illness, its stage, and its location. It's crucial to remember that many symptoms could overlap with several non-cancerous conditions. Additionally, many cancers may not generate apparent symptoms in their early stages. Here is a general discussion of common cancer symptoms:

Unexplained Weight Loss:

Sudden and unexplained weight loss, especially if severe, may be an indication of several cancers. This may occur due to a combination of issues such as loss of appetite and the body's higher energy demands when cancer cells proliferate.

Fatigue:

Persistent, unexplained weariness that doesn't improve with rest may be an indication of numerous malignancies. It may come from the body's immunological response to cancer or the energy needs of the illness.

Pain:

Persistent pain that is not due to an accident or does not improve with usual therapies may be an indication of some malignancies. The pain might vary in severity and location depending on the kind and stage of cancer.

Changes in the Skin:

Skin alterations might include the growth of new moles or changes in existing moles, discoloration, or changes in skin texture. Skin malignancies, such as melanoma, may manifest with obvious abnormalities in the skin.

Changes in Bowel or Bladder Habits:

Persistent changes in bowel habits, such as diarrhea, constipation, blood in the stool, or changes in urine patterns, may be suggestive of colorectal, bladder, or prostate malignancies.

Persistent Cough or Hoarseness:

A persistent cough or hoarseness that does not resolve may be an indication of lung or throat cancer. Blood in the sputum or chronic respiratory difficulties should also be investigated.

Difficulty Swallowing:

Difficulty swallowing or chronic indigestion might be signs of esophageal, stomach, or upper digestive tract malignancies. It may produce pain or a sensation of fullness after a few meals.

Lumps or Swellings:

The development of unexplained lumps or swellings in any region of the body, such as the breasts, testicles, lymph nodes, or beneath the skin, may be symptomatic of malignant growth.

Changes in Bowel or Urinary Habits:

Persistent changes in bowel habits, such as diarrhea or constipation, or changes in urinary patterns, such as increased frequency or blood in the urine, may be indicators of colorectal, bladder, or prostate malignancies.

Fever and Night Sweats:

Persistent, unexplained fevers and night sweats, typically accompanied by other symptoms, may be linked with some forms of malignancies, including lymphomas.

Difficulty Breathing:

Shortness of breath or trouble breathing that is not due to a known respiratory ailment may be a sign of lung or other respiratory system malignancies.

It's crucial to remember that these symptoms may be caused by numerous illnesses, and having them does not always imply cancer. However, if you observe persistent or increasing symptoms, it is vital to speak with a healthcare expert for a comprehensive examination and necessary diagnostic testing. Early identification and therapy dramatically improve results for many forms of cancer.

CHAPTER TWO

Breakfasts for Energy and Vitality

Simple Berry Chia Seed Pudding

The easiest, most personalized, and healthiest breakfast ever.preparation Time is 5 minutes and it's ready in 2-3 hours or overnight!

Prep Time: 5 minutes

Soaking Time: 2 hours Hours

Total Time: 2 Hours 5 minutes

Ingredients

- 1/3 cup chia seeds
- 1 cup unsweetened almond milk, oat milk, or other non-dairy milk
- 1 tsp honey or maple syrup, optional I forego the sweetener, and it tastes amazing!
- a handful of every single freshly picked strawberry and blueberry, for sprinkling

Method Of Preparation

1. Add chia seeds and milk to a mason jar or plate. For a thicker pudding, add 1/3 cup chia seeds. Stir completely and place a lid or plastic wrap over it to cover.

2. Permit pudding to rest for two to three hours or overnight.

3. Whenever the pudding is set, it should be smooth and thick. Stir well and add fresh strawberries and blueberries. If making two servings, divide the pudding between two jars/bowls.

4. Enjoy instantly or store in the fridge for up to 5 days.

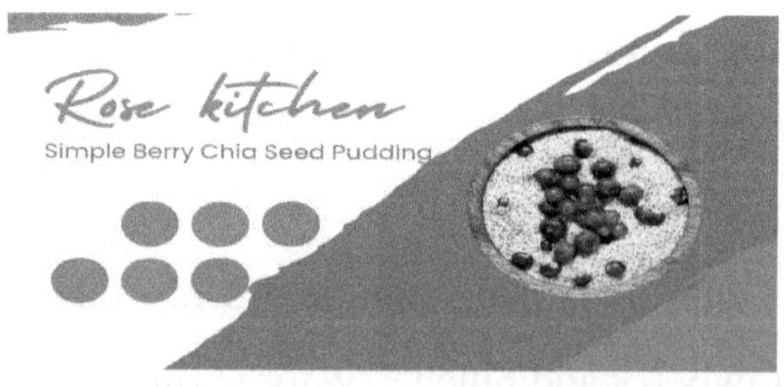

Sweet Potato and Kale Breakfast Hash

Looking for a nice and wholesome meal for Meatless Monday? Get the recipe for this excellent sweet potato and kale hash for breakfast or supper … or for a kids' meal who prefer breakfast for dinner!

Prep Time: 5 minutes

Cook Time: 15 minutes

Total Time: 20 minutes

Serving size: 4

Ingredients

- 2 T. olive oil
- 1 tsp. ground cumin
- 1 tsp. ground coriander
- 1/2 tsp. paprika
- 1/2 tsp. garlic powder
- 1 small red onion, diced
- 2 huge sweet potatoes, diced

- 1 bunch of kale, thinly sliced
- 1 tsp. salt
- 1/2 tsp. pepper 4 eggs cilantro, for garnish

Method of Preparation

1. Heat a big nonstick saucepan over medium heat.

2. Add the olive oil and onion; sauté until the onion is translucent, about 3-4 minutes.

3. Add sweet potatoes and boil until fork tender, about 8 minutes, stirring periodically.

4. Sprinkle sweet potatoes with cumin, coriander, paprika, garlic powder, salt, and pepper and stir until equally coated.

5. Add the kale and cook until just wilted, roughly 2 minutes.

6. To cook the eggs, put the sweet potato and kale mixture into the pan while forming 4 tiny divots.

7. Crack the eggs into each divot.

8. lid with a lid and cook for about 3-4 minutes. We are hoping for the egg whites to harden, while the yolk remains fluid.

9. Just before serving, sprinkle with cilantro.

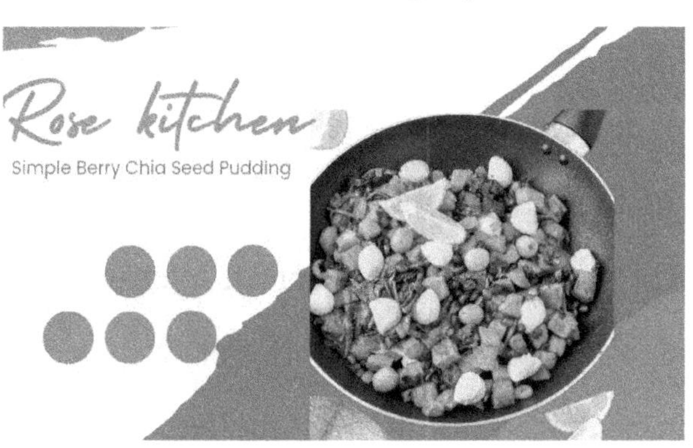

Spinach and Mushroom Omelette

A quick and easy meal, packed with health, this Spinach and Mushroom Omelette is excellent for a simple breakfast or a light dinner

Prep Time: 5 minutes

Cook Time: 5 minutes

Total Time: 10 Minutes

Serving size: 1

Ingredients

- 1 teaspoon butter
- 2 chestnut mushrooms cut thinly
- 1 handful of baby spinach
- 2 big eggs
- 20 g cheddar cheese grated
- Salt and pepper to taste

Method of Preparation

- Set a tiny frying pan over an average heat and add a little bit of butter. When the butter has completely melted add the mushrooms. Sauté the mushrooms for a few moments on each side and then add a small amount of spinach. Stir to help the spinach wilt.

- Meanwhile, break the eggs into a cup or small jug and stir with a fork. Add the

grated cheese, salt, and pepper, and mix to
incorporate.

- Tip the eggs into the pan and swirl quickly
  to combine with the mushrooms and
  spinach. Then let it set until the bottom of
  the omelette is deep brown and the top is
  almost but not quite set.

- Flip the omelette in half and tip out onto a
  platter. Serve with a simple salad and a
  great large slice of crusty French Bread

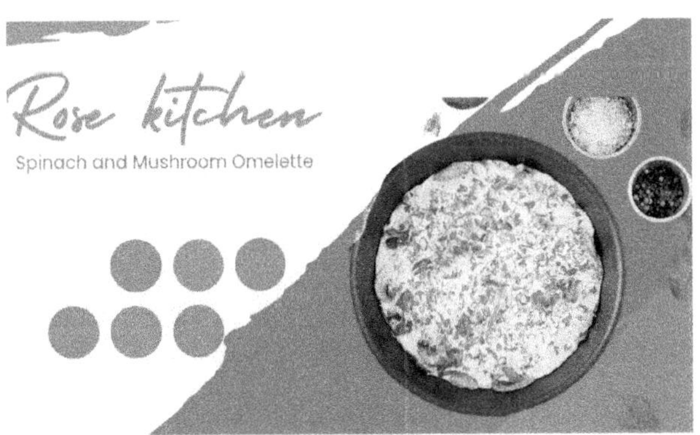

Spinach and Mushroom Omelette

Hot Smoked Salmon & Avocado Breakfast Wraps

A touch of chopping and mashing, a quick stir, a quick squeeze or two and you're ready to roll.

Prep time: 10 minutes

Cook time:

Serves: 2

Ingredients

- 1 ripe avocado
- ½ lemon, juice
- 2 flour tortillas
- 1 hot smoked salmon fillet
- 2 tbsp crème fraiche
- 1 tbsp horseradish
- 1 red onion, thinly sliced
- 2 tbsp fresh dill, chopped

Method of Preparation

1. Mash the avocado with a little squeeze of the lemon and distribute it between the two wraps. Scatter the salmon on top.

2. Stir the fresh crème fraîche with the horseradish and the remainder of the lemon juice. Drizzle over the salmon and avocado. Now distribute over the onion and chopped dill.

3. Sprinkle with salt and pepper, then wrap up the wraps and cut in half.

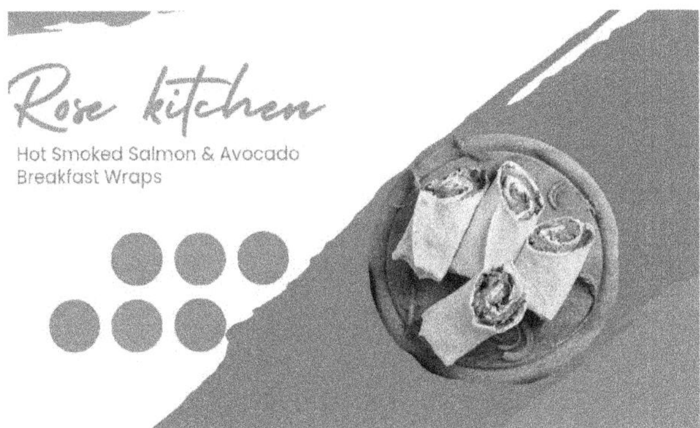

Almond Butter and Banana Smoothie

This banana almond butter smoothie is very easy to make together with just 4 basic ingredients! It's refreshing and certain to be a success with both kids and adults!

Preparation Time: 5 minutes

Total Time: 5 minutes

Servings Size: 2

Ingredients

- 1 cup sugar-free vanilla almond milk
- 1 banana, frozen or fresh
- 1 Tablespoon almond butter
- 4-5 ice cubes

Method of Preparation

1. Add all ingredients to a high-powered blender and mix until smooth.

2. Pour into two glasses and enjoy

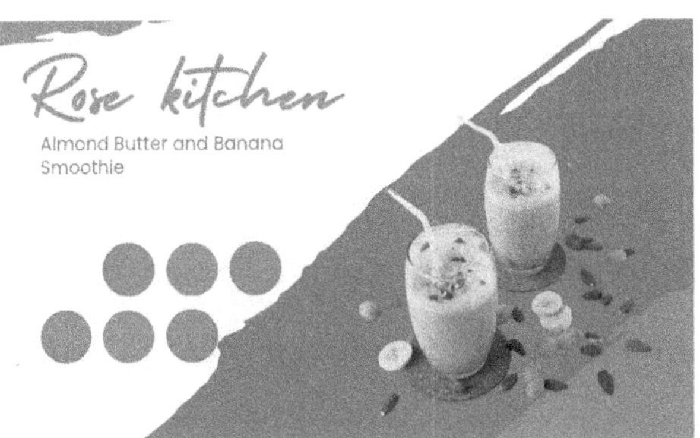

CHAPTER THREE

Lunches for Nourishment

Lentil and Vegetable Soup

This cosy vegetarian lentil soup is packed with goodies - excellent for keeping you warm on cold nights! Learn how to prepare vegetable and red lentil soup with this simple recipe. Simply serve with crusty bread for a hearty winter supper

Preparation Time: 15 Minutes

cooking Time: 37 Minutes

Total Time: 52 Minutes

Serving Size: 2

Ingredients

- 1 onion
- 1 carrot
- 1 leek
- 1 potato

- 2 celery sticks

- 1 tbsp olive oil

- 1 tbsp plain flour

- 1 tsp stock powder

- 500ml boiling water

- 50g red lentils

Method Of Preparation

1. Head and tail the carrot, then peel, cube, and wash it.

2. Also, top and tail the leek, eliminate the outer covering, and then peel, slice, and wash it.

3. Peel and cube the potato. Wash the celery, before chopping it into pieces roughly 2cm in length.

4. Heat the oil in a skillet and sauté all the veggies, except the potatoes, for 5

minutes. Whisk in the flour and sauté for 2 minutes.

5. Mix the stock powder in boiling water, before adding it to the pot and bringing it to the boil.

6. Add the potatoes and red lentils, before placing a cover on the saucepan and leaving all the ingredients to boil for 30 minutes.

7. Serve this rich soup with crusty bread.

8. Tip: You may substitute the leek and carrot with different veggies.

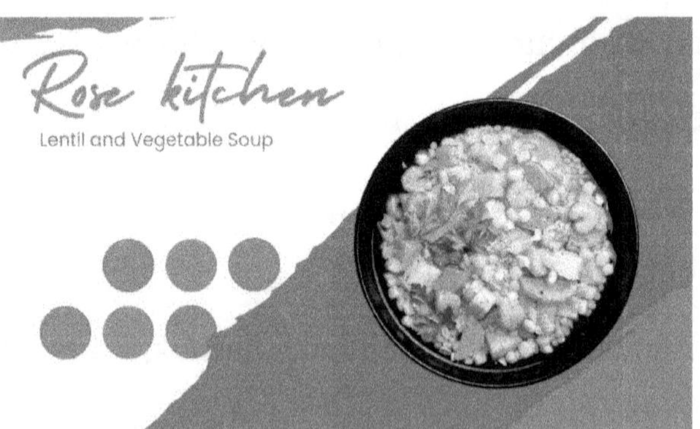

Roasted Vegetable Quinoa Bowls

These quick roasted veggie quinoa bowls are perfect for lunch or supper! They are gluten-free, vegan, and perfect for meal planning. Make it on Sunday and eat all week!

Preparation Time: 20 Minutes

Cooking Time: 40 Minutes

Total Time: 1 Hour

Ingredients

For the vegetables:

- 1 big sweet potato cut into 1/2-inch chunks
- 2 cups broccoli florets
- 2 cups cauliflower florets
- 2 cups Brussels sprouts sliced in half
- 1/2 red onion sliced
- 1-2 tbsp olive oil
- Salt and black pepper to taste

- 3 cups chopped kale

For the Quinoa:

- 1 cup quinoa washed

- 2 cups water

- Pinch of salt

- For the Lemon Tahini Dressing: 1/3 cup tahini

- 1 clove garlic

- 4 tablespoons lemon juice

- 1/3 cup warm water

- Salt and pepper to taste

Method Of Preparation

1. Preheat the oven to 400 degrees F. Place the veggies on two baking pans, ensuring they are in a uniform layer and spread out a bit. Drizzle with olive oil and mix until the veggies are coated. Season with salt

and black pepper. Place in the oven and cook for 20 minutes.

2. Remove from the oven and mix the veggies. Place the pans back in the oven and roast for 15-20 more minutes or until the veggies are soft and slightly crunchy. I want my veggies crispy and a touch black on the edges so I let them roast for about 40 minutes total.

3. While the veggies are roasting prepare the quinoa. In a medium saucepan, add water, rinsed quinoa, and salt. Bring to a boil. Decrease the heat to low and cover with a lid. Sauté for 15 minutes. Withdraw from heat and let stand for 5 minutes, covered. Take out the cover and mix the quinoa using a fork.

4. To create the lemon tahini dressing, mix the tahini, garlic, lemon juice, and water

in a small dish or jar. Season with salt and pepper, to taste. If the covering is too firm, add a bit of extra water and whisk again.

5. To construct the bowls, add quinoa, an array of roasted veggies, and chopped kale. Drizzle with lemon tahini dressing.

6. Note-If you are meal preparing, you may put the dressing in a different container and wait to dress the bowls. You may heat the roasted veggies and quinoa in the microwave and add the greens and dressing when you are ready to eat. Feel free to roast whichever veggies you wish!

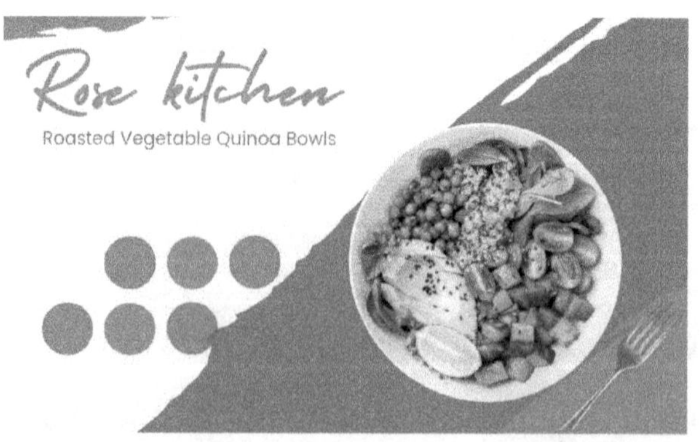

Baked Salmon with Lemon and Dill

Baked Salmon with Lemon and Dill: A delicious meal containing oven-baked salmon flavored with zesty lemon and fragrant dill, creating a beautiful symphony of freshness and richness."

Preparation Time: 10 Minutes

Cooking Time: 15 Minutes

Resting Time: 10 Minutes

Serving Size: 4 persons

Ingredients

- 4 6 oz salmon fillets (we prefer Costco salmon)
- 1 tbsp olive oil salt and spice to taste
- lemon slices for garnish if needed
- Lemon Dill Sauce
- 1/3 cup Greek yogurt
- 2 tbsp mayonnaise

- 1.5 tbsp dill (shredded if using fresh) (we use chill dried but freshly picked is fine too)
- 2 tbsp lemon juice
- 1 tsp lemon zest
- 1 tsp powdered garlic salt and pepper to taste

Method of Preparation

1. Preheat the oven to 400 degrees Fahrenheit.
2. Place fish on a foil-lined baking tray. Sprinkle the top with olive oil, salt and pepper. Cook for 12-16 minutes based on the thickness of the salmon fillet. Once the internal temperature reaches around 135 degrees, remove it from the oven and allow it to rest till 145 degrees inside (the proper cooking point for salmon).

3. While the fish is baking, whisk together the dill sauce ingredients. Set aside.

4. Once the salmon is cooked to your taste, add dill sauce on top. Garnish with lemon wedge if preferred and serve

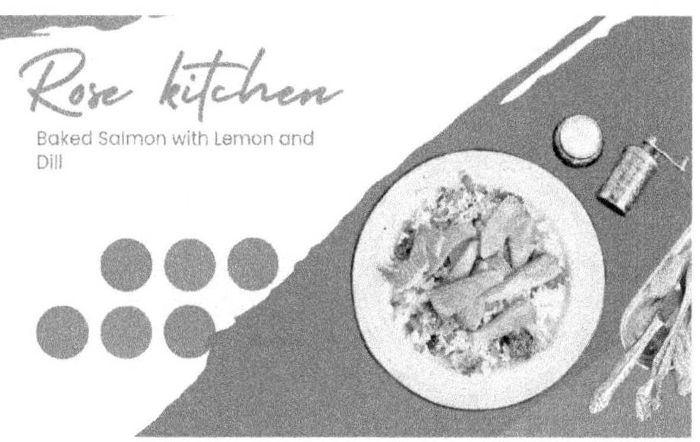

Baked Salmon with Lemon and Dill

Chickpea and Avocado Wrap:

This avocado wrap with chickpeas is ready in only 10 minutes and is excellent for a nutritious meal prep lunch! The fast maple chickpeas combine wonderfully with a mellow avocado sauce, both needing only a handful of ingredients. Gluten-free and oil-free.

Preparation Time: 5 Minutes

Cooking Time: 20 Minutes

Total Time: 25 Minutes

Ingredients

For the chickpeas

- 1 can chickpeas (240g or 1.5 cups)
- 1 tbsp maple syrup
- 1 tsp cumin
- 1 tsp turmeric
- 1 tsp salt

For the avocado sauce

- 1 big avocado mashed

- ½ cup fresh dill chopped

- 2 tbsp tamari

- ½ lemon juice of 3 tbsp soy yogurt

- To serve

- 2 big gluten-free tortillas

Method of Preparation

1. Add the chickpeas, maple sugar, cumin, turmeric, and salt to a non-stick frying pan and heat for 5-6 minutes, flattening down approximately ½ of the chickpeas.

2. Meanwhile, create the avocado sauce by whisking together the avocado mashed up with the fresh dill, tamari, lemon juice, and soy yogurt.

3. Once the chickpeas are cooked, construct the wrap. Spread over a layer of the avocado sauce, followed by the chickpeas.

4. Finish Fold over the edges, then roll up from the bottom edge. Serve it immediately, or store it in the fridge for 2-3 days.

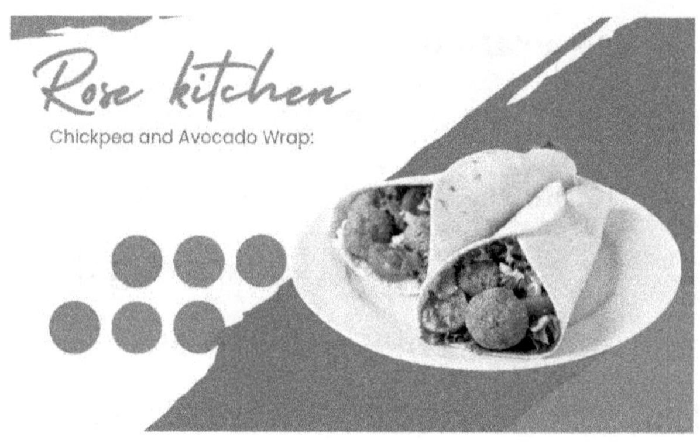

Turmeric broccoli soup

Turmeric Broccoli Soup A vivid and nutritious combination of antioxidant-rich broccoli combined with the warmth of turmeric, producing a cosy soup that delights the palate and enhances general well-being.

Preparation Time: 10 minutes

Cooking Time: 20 minutes

Total Time: 30 minutes

Ingredients

- 1 Tbsp olive oil
- ⅔ cup diced onion
- 2 garlic cloves, minced or crushed
- 1 Tbsp ground turmeric
- 6 cups broccoli florets (and stems)
- 2 cups diced russet potatoes
- 4 cups vegetable or chicken broth
- 1 Tbsp lemon juice

- salt & pepper

Method of Preparation

1. Preheat the oil in a big skillet over moderate heat.

2. Add the onion and simmer for 2 minutes before adding the garlic and turmeric. Cook while stirring for 30 seconds before adding the broccoli and cubed potatoes.

3. Cook the veggies for 2 minutes, stirring regularly, then add the broth.

4. Bring the broth to a boil, and cook with the cover on until all of the veggies are fork-soft (approximately 10 minutes).

5. Use a handheld blender to mix the soup until smooth. Add the lemon juice, and season with a little pepper and salt to taste.

Rose kitchen

Turmeric broccoli soup

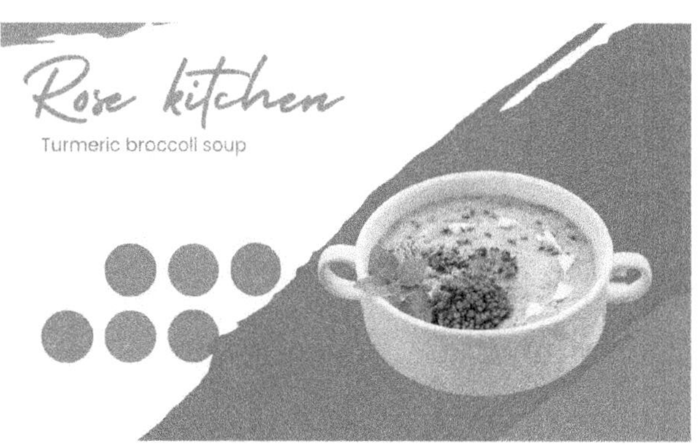

CHAPTER FOUR

Dinners for Comfort and Healing

Baked Cod with Garlic and Herbs

This baked fish is marinated with olive oil, garlic, and fresh herbs, and then roasted to delicate and flaky perfection. A lighter dinner alternative that takes only minutes to put together and is filled with flavor.

Preparation Time: 10 Minutes

Cooking Time: 15 Minutes

Marinating Time: 30 Minutes

Total Time: 55 Minutes

Serving size: 4

Ingredients

- 1 1/4 pounds cod sliced into 4 fillets
- 1/4 cup olive oil
- 2 teaspoons honey
- 1 tablespoon soy sauce

- 3/4 teaspoon lemon zest 2 tablespoons minced fresh parsley + additional for garnish
- 1 1/2 tablespoons fresh thyme leaves
- 1/2 teaspoon salt
- 1/4 teaspoon pepper
- 1 teaspoon minced garlic
- cooking spray
- lemon wedges and fresh herbs for garnish

Method of Preparation

1. In a separate bowl, mix the olive oil, honey, soy sauce, lemon zest, parsley, thyme, salt, pepper, and garlic.

2. Add the fish to the container and ladle the marinade around the top. Cover and leave in the fridge for at least 30 minutes, or as long as eight hours.

3. Prepare the oven to 400 degrees F. Oil a baking dish with the cooking spray.

4. Arrange the fish pieces into the prepared dish. Spoon the marinade over the fish. Oven for 10-11 minutes or until the fish is opaque and slightly cooked through.

5. activate the oven.

6. Saute for 2-4 minutes or until the edges of the fish are golden browned.

7. Serve immediately, topped with fresh herbs and lemon wedges.

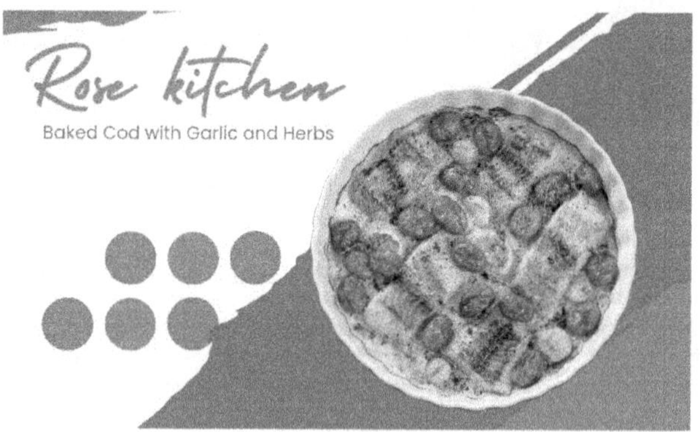

Quinoa Stuffed Bell Peppers

Quinoa Stuffed Bell Peppers: Colourful bell peppers are stuffed with a delightful combination of protein-packed quinoa, colorful veggies, and fragrant spices, delivering a nutritious and pleasant plant-based feast in every bite.

Preparation Time: 20 Minutes

Cooking Time: 30 Minutes

Total Time: 50 Minutes

Ingredients

- 3 cups cooked quinoa
- 1 4-ounce can green chiles
- 1 cup corn kernels
- ½ cup of canned black beans drained and rinsed
- ½ cup tiny chopped tomatoes
- ½ cup shredded pepper jack cheese

- ¼ cup crumbled feta cheese
- 3 tablespoons chopped fresh cilantro leaves
- 1 teaspoon cumin
- 1 teaspoon garlic powder
- ½ teaspoon onion powder
- ½ teaspoon chile powder, or more to taste
- Little Kosher salt and freshly ground black pepper, to taste
- 6 bell peppers, tops chopped, stemmed and seeded

Method of Preparation

1. Warm oven to 350° F. Line a 9×13 baking pan with the parchment paper.
2. In a big container, add quinoa, green chiles, corn, beans, tomatoes, cheeses, cilantro, cumin, garlic, onion and chili powder, salt, and pepper, to taste.

3. Pour the contents into each bell pepper cavity. Place on a prepared baking sheet, cavity side up, and bake until the peppers are soft and the sauce is cooked through approximately 25-30 minutes.

4. Serve immediately.

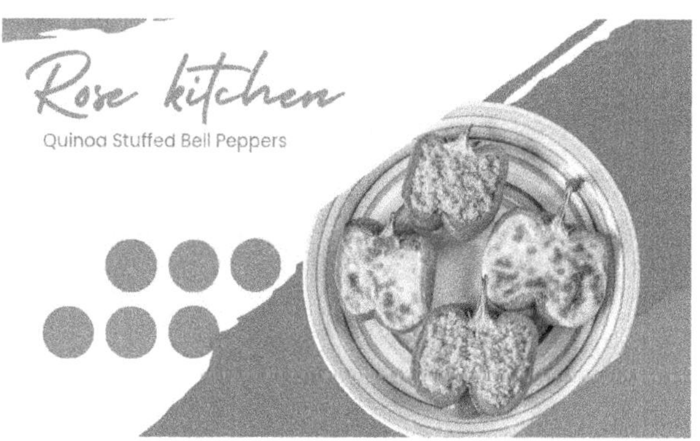

Eggplant and Chickpea Curry

Eggplant meets chickpeas in this vegan, chickpea variant of Baingan Bharta. Spicy, aromatic, and simply amazing! And it's a zero points supper on Weight Watchers!

Preparations Time: 10 Minutes

Cooking Time: 1 Hour 5 Minutes

Total Time: 1 Hour 15 minutes

Servings Size: 4

Ingredients

- 1 huge eggplant
- 1 medium onion, chopped
- 1/2 red bell pepper seeded and chopped
- 1 1/4 teaspoon cumin seeds
- 1 1/4 teaspoon ground coriander
- 1/2 teaspoon turmeric
- 1/8 teaspoon cayenne pepper (or 1 clove garlic, pressed)

- 1 14-ounce can of chopped tomatoes (fire-roasted suggested)
- 2 tablespoons ginger paste or chopped ginger root
- 1/2 teaspoon cayenne or other spicy red pepper (less or more, to taste)
- 1 15-ounce can cooked chickpeas, rinsed and drained (about 1 1/2 cups)
- 1/2 cup water
- 1/4 cup minced parsley or cilantro
- 1/4 teaspoon garam masala (start with less and add more to taste)

Method of Preparation

1. Warm oven to 400F. Prick eggplant with a fork several times and place on a baking pan. Cook for 35-40 minutes, till eggplant is sunken and soft all the way through. Get rid of from oven and set aside until

sufficiently cool to handle. Peel and slice the eggplant flesh.

2. Preheat a non-stick skillet. Add the onion and cook until it begins to turn golden. Add the bell pepper and cook for a few more minutes. Clear a spot in the center of the pan and sprinkle the cumin seeds directly on the hot surface.

3. Stir and roast them for about a minute, until they become fragrant. Stir them into the onions and spicy peppers and add the cilantro, turmeric, asafetida (or garlic), tomatoes, ginger paste, and red pepper.

4. Add the vegetables and simmer over medium heat, pressing eggplant with the back of a spoon to break up large chunks, for roughly 10 minutes. Add the chickpeas and enough water or chickpea cooking

liquid to keep the mixture moist, cover tightly, and decrease the heat to low.

5. Cook for at least 15 minutes, stirring frequently, until sauce has thickened and flavors have blended. (You may leave this dish on low for up to 45 minutes while you prepare the rest of your supper, but add extra liquid as necessary, and don't forget to stir, scraping the bottom.)

6. Just before serving, add cilantro (or parsley), garam masala, and salt to taste. Serve with rice or Indian bread.

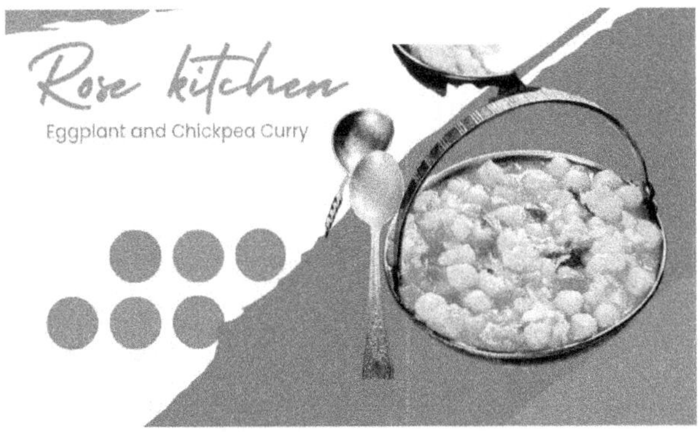

Zucchini Noodles with Pesto

Zucchini Noodles with Pesto: A light and refreshing take on conventional pasta, with zucchini noodles lightly covered in vivid pesto, producing a tasty and healthy meal that's as enjoyable as it is healthful.

Preparation Time: 15 minutes

Total Time: 15 minutes

Serving Size: 4

Ingredients

- 4 tiny zucchini ends clipped
- 2 cups packed fresh basil leaves
- 2 cloves garlic
- 1/3 cup extra-virgin olive oil
- 2 teaspoons fresh lemon juice
- 1/4 cup freshly grated Parmesan cheese
- Kosher salt and powdered black pepper to your liking

- Cherry or grape tomatoes optional

Method of Preparation

1. Use a julienne peeler or mandoline to slice the zucchini into noodles. Set aside.

2. Combine the basil and garlic in a food processor and pulse until roughly chopped. Slowly add the olive oil in a continuous stream while the food processor is on. Stop the machine and scrape down the edges of the food processor with a rubber spatula.

3. Add the lemon juice and Parmesan cheese. Pulse until blended. Season with salt and pepper.

4. Combine the zucchini noodles and pesto. Toss until zucchini noodles are fully coated. Top with tomatoes, if using. Serve at room temperature or cooled.

5. Note-if you want to boil the zucchini noodles, you can. Just add the zucchini pesto noodles to a pan and sauté them over medium heat. It just takes a few minutes.

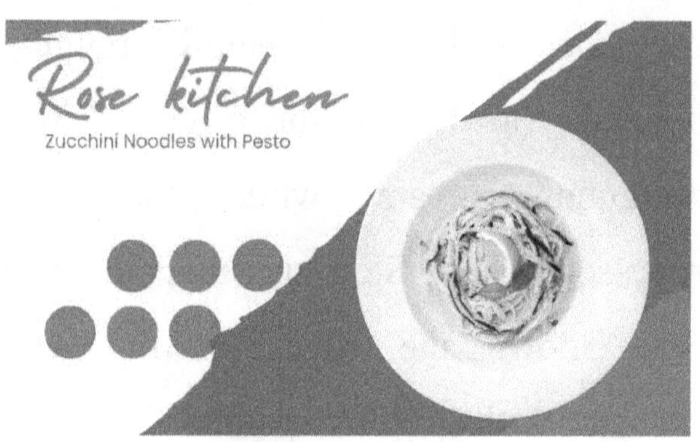

Garlic Roasted Salmon & Brussels Sprouts

Roasting salmon on top of Brussels sprouts and garlic, seasoned with wine and fresh oregano, is easy enough for a weekday supper but elegant enough to serve to guests. Serve with whole-wheat couscous.

Cooking Time: 25 Minutes

Additional Time: 20 Minutes

Total Time: 45 Minutes

Servings Size: 6

Ingredients

- 14 huge cloves garlic, divided
- ¼ cup extra-virgin olive oil
- 2 tablespoons finely chopped fresh oregano, divided
- 1 teaspoon salt,
- ¾ teaspoon freshly ground pepper, divided

- 6 cups Brussels sprouts, trimmed and sliced
- ¾ cup white wine, ideally Chardonnay
- 2 pounds wild-caught salmon fillet, peeled, cut into 6 parts
- Lemon wedges

Method of Preparation

1. Preheat oven to 450 degrees F
2. Mince 2 garlic cloves and put in a small dish with oil, 1 tablespoon oregano, 1/2 teaspoon salt and 1/4 teaspoon pepper.
3. Halve the remaining garlic and combine with Brussels sprouts and 3 tablespoons of the seasoned oil in a large roasting pan. Roast, stirring once, for 15 minutes.
4. Add wine to the remaining oil mixture. Remove the skillet from the oven, toss the veggies, and add fish on top.

5. Drizzle with the wine mixture. garnish with the remainder of 1 tablespoon of oregano and half a teaspoon of salt and pepper. Bake until the salmon is barely cooked through, 5 to 10 minutes longer. Serve with lemon wedges.

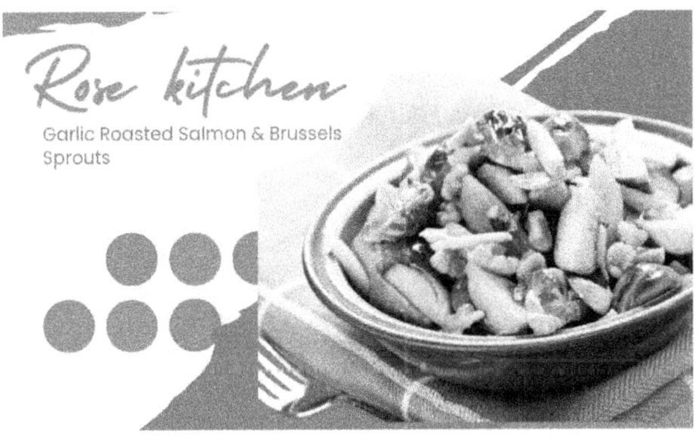

CHAPTER FIVE

Smoothies for Healing

Spinach Berry Smoothie

This Spinach Berry smoothie is wonderful if you're wanting a simple green smoothie. High in fibre and ideal for that midday energy boost.

Preparations Time: 5 Minutes

Total Time: 5 Minutes

Serving Size: 1

Ingredients

- 1 cup spinach
- 1 cup almond milk
- 1 cup mixed berries frozen
- 1 banana
- 1 serving of homemade protein powder optional

Method Of Preparation

1. Place spinach and water in a blender. Puree until smooth.

2. Add fruit and blend again.

3. NOTES Use frozen fruit to generate a delightfully cooled smoothie.

4. To cut down on the natural sugars in this smoothie, substitute 1 banana with 1/2 avocado or 1/2 cup frozen cauliflower.

5. Swap spinach for the leafy greens of your preference.

6. Add a plant-based protein powder for added protein and healthy fat.

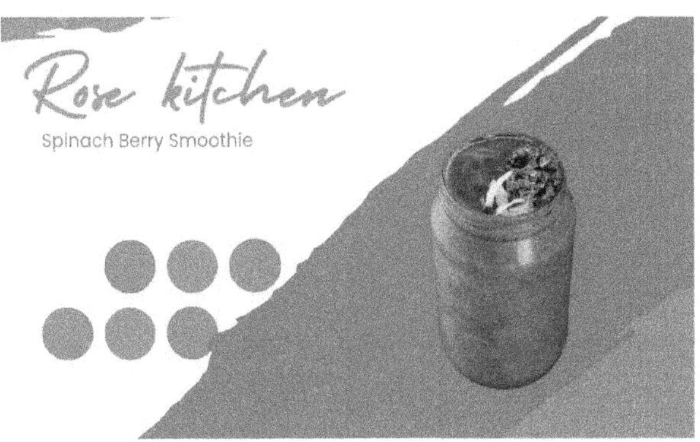

Green Tea and Berry Antioxidant Smoothie

This green tea ginger smoothie is also a wonderful source of antioxidants that fuel our bodies and help battle the adverse environmental conditions we are exposed to in everyday life.

Total Time: 10 Minutes

Servings Size: one 2-1/4 cups smoothie

Ingredients

- ½ cup prepared green tea, room temperature or cold
- 1 teaspoon coconut oil
- 1 teaspoon peeled and sliced fresh ginger
- 2 huge kale leaves, cut from the stem (chopped if required for your blender model)
- 1 cup fresh blueberries, rinsed
- ½ cup golden colour or red raspberries, either fresh or frozen

- Optional: 1 teaspoon chia seeds

Method Of Preparation

1. Mix all of the ingredients in an immersion blender and pulse until creamy and smooth. Enjoy!

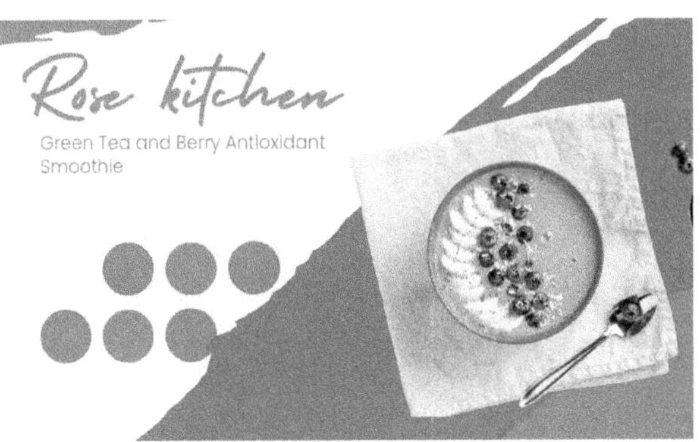

Pineapple Turmeric Ginger Elixir

This Pineapple Turmeric Ginger Elixir is a healthy drink that's just as delightful as it is wonderful for you. Pineapple juice, ginger beer, turmeric, and fresh lime blend to produce a wonderful drink that's ideal for summer!

Preparations Time: 5 Minutes

Total Time: 5 Minutes

Servings: 2

Ingredients

- Ice

- 1/2 teaspoon ground turmeric

- 4 ounces pineapple juice (no sugar added if practical)

- Juice of 1/2 a lime

- 4 ounces of ginger beer

- Lime wheels or wedges for garnish

Method Of Preparation

1. Fill in a cocktail shaker half full with ice, then add turmeric, pineapple juice, and lime. Mix continuously for 10-15 seconds.

2. Fill a pair of rock glasses with ice and strain the contents of the cocktail shaker evenly between the two.

3. Topped with ginger wine and sprinkled with lime wheels or wedges.

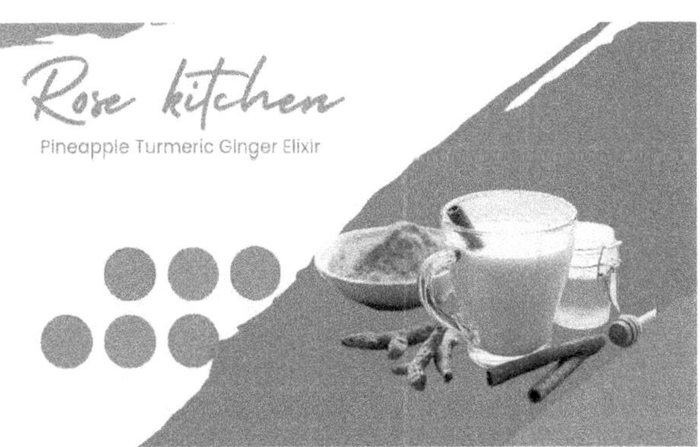

Pineapple Turmeric Ginger Elixir

Avocado And Mint Green Smoothie

Creamy avocado, fresh spinach, and mint are the stars of this delicious green smoothie filled with health-giving benefits.

Preparations Time: 5 Minutes

Total Time: 5 Minutes

Serving Size: 1

Ingredients

- ½ a ripe avocado
- 1 over-ripe banana fresh or frozen
- 1 cup spinach leaves (approximately 3-4 large leaves or a huge handful of baby spinach)
- ½ cup fresh mint leaves
- Juice of one lime (approximately 2 tbsp)
- ½ cup almond milk or water

Method Of Preparation

1. Put all ingredients into a blender, and mix until smooth.

2. If you want your smoothies extremely chilly, use frozen banana, or add a few ice cubes (and a bit less almond milk to make up for the additional liquid).

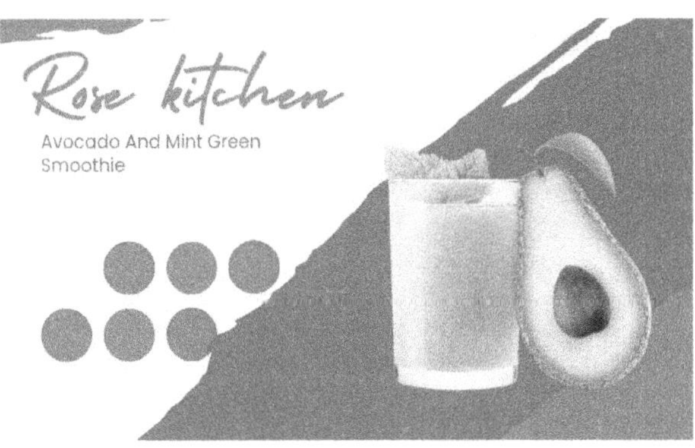

Watermelon and cucumber cooler

This thirst-quenching cooler is a fantastic summer refreshment that will chill you down in the most delightful manner imaginable! The mix of juicy watermelon and crisp cucumber offers a delicious taste that's accentuated by a dash of lime and a touch of sweetness.

Preparation Time: 30 Minutes

Serving Size: 1

Ingredients

- 1 cup sugar(200 g)
- 1 cup water(240 mL)
- 1 cucumber, sliced ice
- 2 oz gin(60 mL)
- 1 ½ ounce watermelon(45 mL), juiced
- ½ ounce lime juice(15 mL)
- 1 oz cucumber simple syrup(30 mL)
- club soda, to taste

- 1 slice cucumber, for garnish

Method of Preparation

1. In a little saucepan over moderate heat, mix the sugar in it and water. Bring to a boil, stirring to dissolve the sugar fully.

2. Remove the saucepan from the heat and whisk in the cucumber. Let high, covered up, for a minimum of 4 hours or up to overnight.

3. Strain the syrup through a fine-mesh strainer or cheesecloth, pressing to extract as much syrup as possible. Maintain an airtight jar in the fridge for one month.

4. In a cocktail shaker packed with ice, add the gin, watermelon juice, lime juice, and simple syrup. Shake vigorously for twenty seconds.

5. Pour into a glass filled with ice and top with clubs soda.

6. Garnish with the cucumber slice.

7. Enjoy!

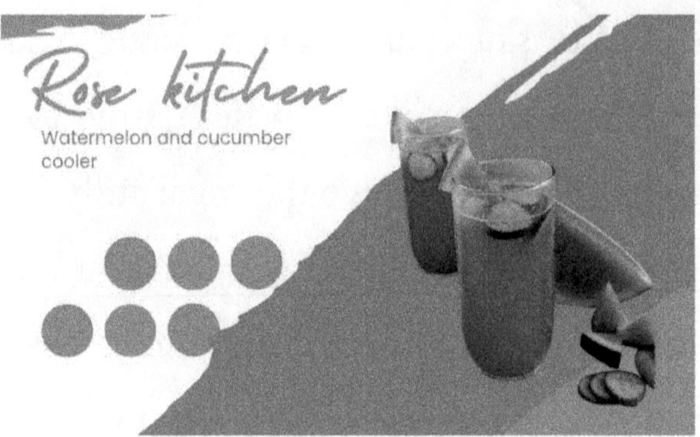

CHAPTER SIX

Snacks and Treats for Sustained Energy

Garlic Mashed Cauliflower

These cauliflower "mashed potatoes" are the ideal low-carb side dish. When I began the South Beach Diet, I couldn't eat mashed potatoes and this dish was a wonderful replacement. Even folks who loathe veggies adore it! I do suggest using a big food processor for this recipe.

Preparation Time: 15 Minutes

Cook Time: 10 Minutes

Total Time: 25 minutes

Servings: 4

Ingredients

- 1 head cauliflower, cut into florets
- 1 tablespoon olive oil
- 1 clove garlic, smashed
- ¼ cup grated Parmesan cheese

- 1 tablespoon reduced-fat cream cheese

- ½ teaspoon kosher salt

- ⅛ teaspoon freshly ground black pepper

Method of Preparation

1. Put a steamer insert into a skillet; fill it with water approximately below the bottom of the boiler. Bring water to a boil; add cauliflower, cover, and steam until tender, approximately 10 minutes.

2. Meanwhile, heat olive oil in a small pan over medium heat; sauté and stir garlic until softened approximately 2 minutes. Remove from heat.

3. Transfer 1/2 of the cauliflower to a food processor; cover and mix on high. Add remaining cauliflower florets, one at a time, until veggies are creamy.

4. Blend in sautéed garlic, Parmesan cheese, cream cheese, salt, and black pepper.

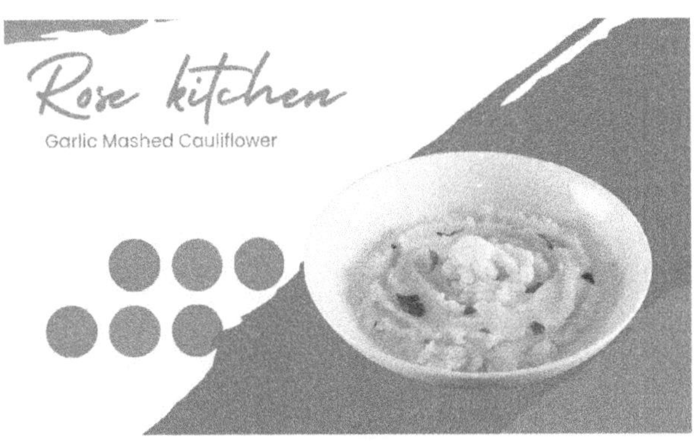

Avocado And Tomato Salsa

A simple chopped avocado, tomato, red onion, and cilantro salsa seasoned with olive oil, lime, salt, and pepper. This flavour-packed salsa is fantastic over tacos, burrito bowls, grilled meat, or just with tortilla chips.

Preparation Time: 10 Minutes

Total Time: 15 Minutes

Serving Size: 4

Ingredients

- 2 ripe avocados, pitted and diced
- 1 cup tomato, diced (any variety of tomato)
- 1/4 cup onion, chopped
- 1/4 cup cilantro, minced
- 2 tablespoons olive oil
- Zest 1 lime, 2-3 tablespoons salt and pepper, to enjoy

Method of Preparation

1. Add the flesh of the avocado, tomato, onion, and cilantro to a big stirring bowl.

2. Drizzle with olive oil, fresh lime juice, and a bit of salt and pepper. Gently whisk with a spoon until thoroughly blends.

3. Serve immediately or securely cover with plastic wrap and refrigerate for up to 2

days. The lime will protect the avocado from browning.

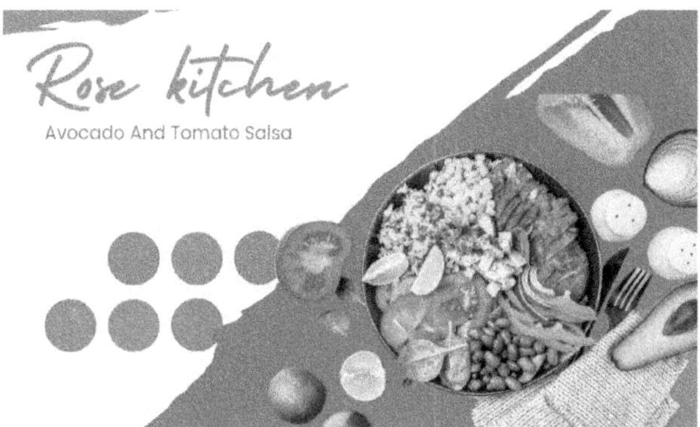

Garlic And Herb Roasted Mushrooms

Mushrooms have a wonderfully meaty texture and these Roasted Garlic and Herb Mushrooms take on the taste of the herbs to form an easy, excellent side dish.

Preparations Time: 5 Minutes

Cooking Time: 15 Minutes

Total Time: 20 Minutes

Serving Size: 2

Ingredients

- 18 Fresh mushrooms - we chose a blend of white and chestnuts
- 3 Garlic clove - crushed 4 tablespoons Fresh parsley - chopped
- 1 sprinkle Sea salt and black pepper
- 2 tbsp Olive oil

Method of Preparation

1. Preheat your oven to 200°C/180°C(fan)/400°F/Gas 6. Quarter 18 Fresh mushrooms and place in a bowl with 3 Garlic cloves, 4 tablespoons Fresh parsley, 2 tablespoons Olive oil, and 1 teaspoon Sea salt and black pepper and combine well.

2. Put on a baking tray.

3. Put into the oven for 15 minutes

4. Then Enjoy

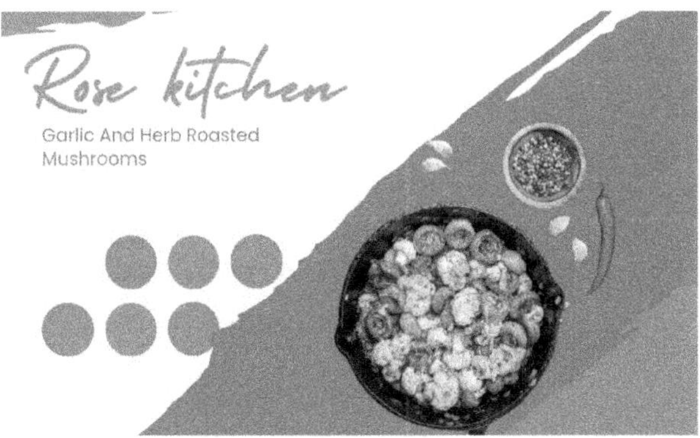

Roasted Asparagus with Balsamic Glaze

Roasted Asparagus with Balsamic Glaze: Tender asparagus stalks, properly roasted to highlight their natural sweetness, drizzled with a magnificent balsamic sauce, providing a delightful side dish that balances earthy notes with a touch of acidic richness.

Preparations Time: 5 Minutes

Cooking Time: 25 Minutes

Total Time: 30 Minutes

Serving Size: 4-6

Ingredients

- 1 cup balsamic vinegar
- 2 tablespoons brown sugar (optional)
- A bunch of thin asparagus, trimmed
- 1 tablespoon olive oil
- 1 teaspoon salt
- 1 teaspoon black pepper

- 1/2 cup shredded Parmesan cheese

Method of Preparation

1. Preheat the oven to 425°.

2. In a small saucepan, bring the balsamic vinegar (and brown sugar, if using) to a boil over medium heat. Once it reaches a gentle boil drop the heat to medium-low and let it simmer, stirring frequently. The vinegar will thicken as it decreases, roughly 20 minutes. The similarity should be sufficiently thick to coat the backside of a spoon.

3. Remove the balsamic glaze from the heat and let it cool thoroughly.

4. Wash off the asparagus leaves and arrange them on a baking tray. Drizzle the oil over the asparagus and then season with salt and pepper.

5. Sprinkle the shredded cheese on top of the asparagus and bake for 15 minutes or until it reaches your ideal tenderness.

6. Once you remove the asparagus from the oven pour the balsamic glaze over the asparagus and enjoy!

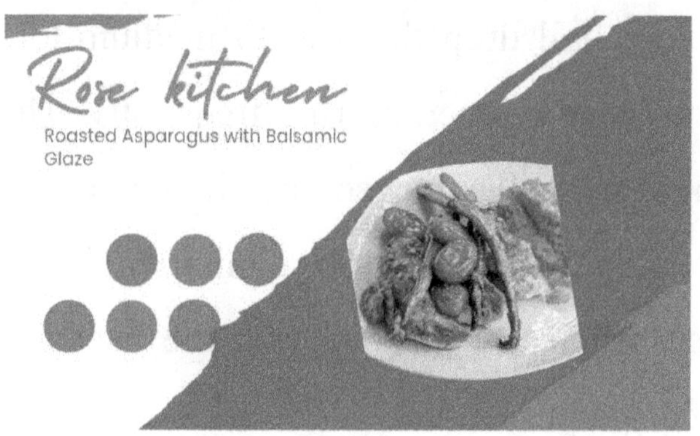

Grilled Eggplant with Tahini Sauce

Grilled Eggplant with Tahini Sauce: Smoky and delicious grilled eggplant slices, artfully complemented with a silky tahini sauce, offering a balanced blend of savory sensations and creamy pleasure in every exquisite mouthful.

Preparations Time: 10 Minutes

Cooking Time: 10 Minutes

Total: 20 Minutes

Serving Size: 4

Ingredients

- 1 eggplant (sliced into thick rounds)
- 2 tablespoons super virgin olive oil with a pinch of pepper (to taste)
- minced fresh parsley or mint (optional garnish)
- Tahini Sauce
- ¼ cup tahini
- 1 tablespoon lemon juice
- 2 tablespoons warm water (or more, to thin)
- ½ teaspoon salt
- 1 clove garlic (minced)
- 1 pinch cayenne (optional)

Method of Preparation

- Preheat the grill to high heat and coat both sides of the eggplant with olive oil. Sprinkle with salt and pepper to taste then grill until done, about 4-5 minutes per side, turning twice on each side before flipping.

- While eggplant is cooking, whisk together tahini sauce in a small basin.

- Remove the eggplant from the grill and place on a platter. Serve eggplant cooked with tahini sauce sprinkled on top. Sprinkle with new mint or parsley if you wish.

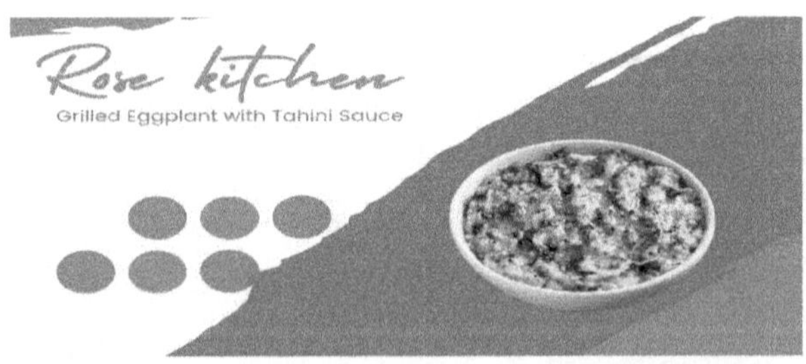

CHAPTER SEVEN

A 7-Day Meal Plan

This specially curated 7-day meal plan is designed with your well-being in mind, embracing nutrient-rich and cancer-friendly ingredients. Packed with antioxidants, lean proteins, and inflammation-fighting foods, each dish aims to nourish and support your health journey. From comforting soups to vibrant smoothies and wholesome wraps, these meals prioritize taste without compromising on nutrition. Remember, dietary choices can play a crucial role in your overall wellness. Consult with your healthcare team and enjoy these delicious recipes as a part of your path to strength and vitality.

Day 1:

Breakfast: Simple Berry Chia Seed Pudding

Lunch: Lentil and Vegetable Soup

Dinner: Baked Cod with Garlic and Herbs

Smoothie: Spinach Berry Smoothie

Side Dish: Garlic Mashed Cauliflower

Day 2:

Breakfast: Sweet Potato and Kale Breakfast Hash

Lunch: Roasted Vegetable Quinoa Bowls

Dinner: Quinoa Stuffed Bell Peppers

Smoothie: Green Tea and Berry Antioxidant Smoothie

Side Dish: Avocado and Tomato Salsa

Day 3:

Breakfast: Spinach and Mushroom Omelette

Lunch: Baked Salmon with Lemon and Dill

Dinner: Eggplant and Chickpea Curry

Smoothie: Pineapple Turmeric Ginger Elixir

Side Dish: Garlic and Herb Roasted Mushrooms

Day 4:

Breakfast: Almond Butter and Banana Smoothie

Lunch: Chickpea and Avocado Wrap

Dinner: Zucchini Noodles with Pesto

Smoothie: Avocado and Mint Green Smoothie

Side Dish: Roasted Asparagus with Balsamic Glaze

Day 5:

Breakfast: Hot Smoked Salmon & Avocado Breakfast Wraps

Lunch: Turmeric Broccoli Soup

Dinner: Garlic Roasted Salmon & Brussels Sprouts

Smoothie: Watermelon and Cucumber Cooler

Side Dish: Grilled Eggplant with Tahini Sauce

Day 6:

Breakfast: Simple Berry Chia Seed Pudding

Lunch: Lentil and Vegetable Soup

Dinner: Baked Cod with Garlic and Herbs

Smoothie: Spinach Berry Smoothie

Side Dish: Garlic Mashed Cauliflower

Day 7:

Breakfast: Sweet Potato and Kale Breakfast Hash

Lunch: Roasted Vegetable Quinoa Bowls

Dinner: Quinoa Stuffed Bell Peppers

Smoothie: Green Tea and Berry Antioxidant Smoothie

Side Dish: Avocado and Tomato Salsa

Here in this wisdom-filled chapter, we have included the opinions of nutritionists, holistic health specialists, and medical doctors to help you find your way to complete wellness.

We provide more than just recipes in "Sowing Wisdom," a complex tapestry of thoughts meant to deepen your knowledge and provide you with the tools you need on your path.

Views from the Profession:

Enter the domain of knowledge as seasoned medical experts discuss the link between cancer and poor diet. The advice of experts in the field, such as oncologists and nutritionists, may illuminate the complex relationship between food and health. The healing process may be approached with more knowledge and agency with the help of each pearl of wisdom.

Holistic Health in Harmony:

This section delves into the complex interplay of the mind, body, and spirit, going beyond the usual to do so. Mental health has a significant effect on one's physical health, and holistic health professionals provide their insight to clarify this relationship. Learn how maintaining a positive mentality may become a vital part of your recovery path, producing a symphony of well-being that reverberates through every chapter of your life.

The Math Behind the Dish:

Embark on a journey exploring the science behind the items on your plate. Nutritionists investigate the nutritional characteristics of essential components in our recipes, revealing the healing potential inside each mouthful. This part is not simply a lesson in cooking; it's a masterclass in the science of feeding, allowing you to make choices that connect with your body's specific requirements.

Practical Tips for Everyday Wellness:

Holistic living is not just for exceptional events; it's a daily practice. Here, professionals share practical strategies for effectively incorporating health into your regular life. From simple rituals to mindful practices, these ideas become weapons in your armory for prolonged well-being, emphasising the concept that every day is a chance for healing.

Balancing Act - Integrating Medical and Holistic Approaches:

Discover the delicate balance between medical treatments and natural alternatives. Experts explain techniques for effortlessly combining both worlds, producing a unified and thorough rehabilitation strategy. This section offers a guide, to navigating the complicated dance between medical science and holistic health to ensure you receive the support you need at every stage.

Sustaining Positivity Through Challenges:

Cancer is a journey filled with hurdles, and having a positive mindset is a great ally. Holistic health professionals provide ways to preserve positivity, giving a toolset to traverse the emotional landscape with strength and grace. This is more than advice; it's a companion guide for finding light in the midst of hardship.

In "Sowing Wisdom," Chapter 4 is not simply a compilation of professional suggestions; it's a symposium of information, a gathering of minds geared at improving your path. As you explore into these pages, absorb the thoughts, and allow the combined knowledge of professionals to be a source of empowerment and enlightenment on your road to holistic recovery.

CONCLUSION

Harvesting Hope - A Culmination of Your Healing Journey

As you open the last pages of "The Ultimate Cancer Diet Cookbook for Newly Diagnosed Individuals," we urge you to bask in the warmth of a conclusion that transcends words on paper. This is not simply an ending; it's a celebration of your strength, a culmination of the knowledge shared, and a beacon of hope illuminating the path to a future full of health and vitality.

In these final moments, we send our deepest congratulations on reaching this milestone in your journey. Your dedication to embracing the transforming power of diet and holistic treatment is remarkable, and we stand by you in admiration of the fortitude you've displayed.

Pause for a minute of thought. Consider the recipes you've investigated, the thoughts you've received, and the trips you've gone on. This is not just a cookbook; it's a tribute to your dedication to well-being and a concrete reminder that every decision you make in your kitchen is a step towards a better, happier you.

As we say goodbye to the cookbook, we want to underline that our journey doesn't stop here. Connect with the author, share your tales, and be a part of a community that celebrates accomplishments, large and small. Your stories add to the collective story of strength and hope that we continue to construct together.

Gratitude permeates these pages as we offer our sincere appreciation for allowing us to be a part of your recovery path. The faith you put in this cookbook is humbling, and we hope it has been a source of inspiration and comfort while you negotiated the challenges of a cancer diagnosis.

Look forward with a vision inspired by optimism. This conclusion is not an ending but a transition—a bridge to the next chapter of your life, where health, happiness, and wonderful meals await. The recipes inside these pages are more than ingredients; they are tools for building a future teeming with well-being.

The last invitation is to continue the discussion. Share your experiences, ideas, and newfound knowledge with others. Your path is unique, and your voice adds dimension to the collective tale of victory over adversity. Together, we form a community of support and understanding that stretches well beyond the bounds of these pages.

In the conclusion of "The Ultimate Cancer Diet Cookbook," we celebrate not only the end of a book but the beginning of a new chapter in your life—one filled with health, healing, and the delight of relishing each moment. May your kitchen continue to be a place of sustenance, your heart a refuge of hope, and your future a canvas painted with the brilliant hues of well-being. Cheers to your trip, and may it be as rich and gratifying as the dishes presented on these pages.